About the author

Dianne Corbeau's writing reflects the internal and external.

Internally, the backstories are woven throughout all her books, revealing her inner process.

Externally, the raw prose in her narrative encapsulates her experience as if you were taking the journey with her.

Dianne continues to write and live out her experience in Cape Cod, Massachusetts.

16 STORIES ABOUT 16 THERAPISTS

Dianne Corbeau

16 STORIES ABOUT 16 THERAPISTS

Vanguard Press

A CIP catalogue record for this title is available from the British
Library.

ISBN 978-1-80016-787-2

Vanguard Press is an imprint of
Pegasus Elliot Mackenzie Publishers Ltd.
www.pegasuspublishers.com

First Published in 2025

Vanguard Press
Sheraton House Castle Park
Cambridge England
Printed & Bound in Great Britain

Dedication

This book is dedicated to Patricia…

Acknowledgements

In acknowledgement of the individuals who believed in me when there was just a shred—A Shred.
It takes one person to believe in the Last Shred.

SYNOPSIS

This manuscript is a complement of sixteen stories based on the research I have done throughout my years to find a therapist. Some did not go so well, others worse, while others saved my life at the time. This relentless read has a fast tempo but a fine thread into each story leading to the next interaction with the previous therapist. The sense of humor is driven in this book and comes up when you least expect it.

It is a truthful, fun, sad, and adventurous read from start to finish.

1st Therapist
A Wolf in Sheep's Clothing

Fourteen years of age, fresh off the streets, surviving in New York City. Introduced to a therapist named Milton by one of my elder friends. The season of summer was always hot, and now, I wearing next to nothing. My first appointment with, 'Old hard on Mil', I was not so sweet sixteen.

Milton was a social worker. In addition, I was fresh off the streets from New York City. He was a quiet-spoken, African American, timid, and slender male. His actions reminded me of a mute goat.

I was introduced to him on a silver platter, from his boss, Carrie. She approached his desk, pointed her finger at my thin beige file and murmured somethings about me, in which I could not tell what they were speaking. Seeing Milton nodding his head up and down with his hand over his mouth and squirming in his skin, as he backed up to speak to Carrie.

Carrie was a wide-legged woman who spent too much time on her butt not caring, handed me over to Milton to his silver platter.

She introduced us, "Milton this is Dianne. Dianne this is Milton, your new counselor."

Simultaneously, Milton and I said, "Hello."

We shook each other's hand as if I could feel the sharpness of his fingertips glide coldly into my palm. I questioned his nervousness but continued to ignore my street smarts and move ahead with this process, thinking, *just maybe this counseling will bring some relief to my painful existence.*

Carrie snapped me out of my frozen trance by saying, "Okay. Let me know if any of you need anything. I will be right down the hall."

Then she turned away and walked in her creaky shoes.

Afterwards, Milton and I glanced at each other as his spidery fingertips pointed me to the direction of the couch.

As soft spoken as he could, he said, "Please, Dianne, have a seat wherever you are comfortable.

The pretend, carefree-step of my young, attractive, slender body slid my way onto the patients' couch.

Like clockwork, Milton took his assigned seat; it was an old-tattered chair, as he brought a note pad and a pen. This was my first time doing this and I noticed that as he asked me questions, I began to be my straightforward self and tell him what I knew to be true and to the point. I began with a true story I remembered; a large, male hand possessed my infant body my body. Just a flash. That was all I would see. As clear as a motion picture but just a four-second flash.

Continuing to answer his questions, I noticed that he crossed his legs as he stroked his hand over his purple lips. Milton's actions seemed off-putting to say the least.

Not knowing what do, I figured, buying time was the only thing that I could do. Now I was squirming in *my* seat, moving closer to the arm of the couch. I told myself not to look down at the couch, as I would be sorry, if I were to look directly at Milton. Even though, I felt the familiar groping feeling in the pit-of-my-stomach, I convinced myself it was my fault and tried to tell him more about my life on the streets in New York City.

Suddenly, I became angry, and told myself to turn-the-tables on him. With all my willpower, I stood my ground.

Then Milton sheepishly stated, "Dianne, let's go back and tell me more about your childhood."

I replied, "Well, I did not feel good about it and it made me feel dirty."

Then I glanced down to the hard on that was in full-salute mode.

With mixed feelings, none of them good, my emotions went on the defense as I could tell he was desperately trying to hold this massive monster back and go unnoticed.

I thought, *not a chance*. It is time for me to make *him* uncomfortable.

Now I was to begin to bring up my up-to-date drug abuse among other street-smart ideas that I needed to protect myself. Not to mention the weapon I had in my back pocket and another one in my shoes.

Nonchalantly, I said to Milton, "I can protect myself."

His eyebrows rose as he looked at me with shock and amazement. The hard-on ceased, but again arose. Vigorously.

Making him embarrassed was my ideal of now being pissed-off and took advantage.

Ever so subtle, I asked Milton, "Where are *you* from?"

We both squirmed, as his hard-on was getting lower. Then it would make his way back up.

He responded, "The Bronx." In addition, continued, "Right down the street… you know?"

My reply was, "Yes, I do know. Moreover, I asked, "Did you grow up poor?'

Confused he was still powerless, inexperienced enough, and gross enough, not to rock the boat.

He answered, "Yes, very much so… I am one of eight children."

Maybe he thought we were bonding, but at this point, I had him, and his hard on in control.

At least I thought.

He gained some sort of clue and brought the conversation to follow-up on me.

He asked, "So, how are you feeling, Dianne?"

Now I was looking at a full-blown hard-on. I thought, *Unbelievable, this person never stops.*

Instead of playing any more games as my eyes glanced back up at his face, he gave me a weird, cold hard stare, not mean, but seemingly dissociated himself.

I looked at the clock behind him and not letting him on of my findings about my diagnosis and his personality traits, was another predator, I said, "I feel good, okay, better. Thank You."

Not being able to wait another minute for him to conclude this ridiculous session.

I jumped out of my seat and said, "Okay, it is time to go!"

Trying not to look all too happy; I did not smile and I looked at him for his reply.

My guess is he had to wait for his hard-on to go down. He uncrossed his locked-legs and brushed his lips again as if he were in deep, pedophile, thought.

He slowly, stood up, and asked me, "Would you like the same time next week, Dianne?"

Immediately I replied with a quick, "Yes."

Then he turned his back on me, while saying, "Well let me write down an appointment card for next week."

Again, as slow as molasses, Milton wrote out the appointment card, and by no means was I keeping the next appointment or him as a counselor.

When he made his slow gestured way to turn around back to face me and hand me his card.

Confronted, by his long-spiderlike fingernails to me, handed me his card.

I took the card with every cell and quickness of my body to get away from him before he could do even something more inappropriate.

By the time, his words came out, "I will see you next week here at the same time, Dianne. Then ended with a question, "Okay, Dianne?'

As my legs began to move myself out the door, I replied, "Yes, see you next week."

Then I led myself out the door and away for the grips of the, 'Trusted, Predator, Milton'.

2nd Therapist
The Face Off.

Immersed in my own pain, which was driving me to the brink of insanity. Still, able to see this therapist's insecurities.

Her name was Dylan. She led me into her room pretending to have all the male energy she needed to handle a 'case' like mine. The room was crowded with weak decor and shrouded in microscopic details of bullshit. Kind of like her. She did not mean what she said because she was lost in her identity as well.

I took the single most uncomfortable, cheap, seat Dylan herself could have invented.

It began... The Face off.

Already, I had looked at her, in contempt.

Without hesitation, and a lot of worry she introduced herself, "Hello Dianne, I am Dylan... Welcome."

Although her undertone was shaped more like a question mark. I looked at her as if she just walked into *my* room and invaded *my* space.

With disregards, and quite affirming, I answered, "Hello."

Then crossed my arms and legs, so there was no way she was breaking through.

Not looking for an emotion or anything resembling a facial expression or beyond the least bit of care. I was done before I got started. I did not like her.

I felt her uncomfortably and in a bit of whimsy she had held. For her to be able to understand me let alone my life would be the most impossible feat.

She was basic, standard, and on an intimate level would never be able to delve deeply on all levels of commitment to my recovery as a human being. Maybe I was too far gone… I do not know.

Next, I glided along the Freudian seat. Obviously, this chair was for her. As she was indirect in her approach, and passive aggressive in her delivery, it made me resent her even more so, which in turn, boiled my blood.

Clearly, we were not a match made in any type of atmosphere. Immediately, I felt this, she would take a too much time just to catch up.

Dr. Dylan Rut resembled her whole name as she made it clear with her non-verbal disrespect—I gave her. Dr. Dylan was clear that I was merely a non-human subtype. Already, the decision was completed and the line was drawn in the sand on both sides.

I would not speak. Instead, I examined *her* and *her* surroundings.

She started to reach for her static memo pad. As my limbs squeezed tighter to my internal organs. Dr. Rut continued by picking up her stationary pen, with her logo and all.

My unapproved look at her up and down. When my eyes made it back to her doe-eyed stare. I lingered my eyes into the pools of the unsatisfactory grade she gave me, by her judgement and the way our session was going.

Here lies were the basic version of the questions she had for me. They already made up unlike our insurance meeting.

Seeing I was not happy, she went ahead and asked me her pre-questioner anyway.

Trying to start at both of us onto her notes, Dr. Dylan asked, "Dianne, how old are you?"

Without reverence, I snapped an answer, "Sixteen."

Again, she continued, through my disapproval, "Are you having any specific issues that are coming up?"

Rolling my eyes, and not giving her the satisfaction, as I did Milton, I flat lined and said, "No, I do not."

Proving again, stopping Dr. D. in her tracks, I could tell she was in a huff and ready to throw the pen down.

She knew it was time to surrender the white flag, and look me in the eyes with the first honest voice and said, "Dianne, you don't want to be here, do you?"

"No." Blank stare. Blank Statement. In addition, me wanting nothing more to get back and blank myself out and paint on a Blank canvas. This is what I lived for, this is what I dreamed for, and above all, my time here was wasted.

Dr. PhD. acknowledged my rudeness and met me halfway, by saying, "Okay, Dianne, you are free to leave."

Without any further notice, I grabbed my handbag, which weighed about a pharmaceutical, one-hundred pounds. I stood straight up and abruptly walked out of her fake room.

When I reached the streets of New York City, I thought, *great now I can take in some real air.*

3rd Therapist
Princeton Joseph

It had been three years before seeing another therapist. This time I graduated to a psychiatrist. His name was Joseph Goldstein. He was a broad, wide man to say the least, weighing in at over four-hundred pounds. Which I find nothing wrong with, except when he begin to preach at me, and speak at me about gaining weight, which was something I was not at all willing to overcome.

The beginning of his prescription pad treatment plan—Haldol, Lithium, Mellaril, Thorazine, Wellbutrin, and others—for starters.

After the mental hospital and detox they sent me to Dr. Goldstein, for even more evaluation, and as my weekly check-in psychiatrist.

Princeton Joseph was always in a three-piece suit and sweating profusely. I would sit there in the leather, murdered, cow-chair as he sat behind his enormous, protective desk. If I complained of one thing, there his hand scribbled to write another scrip, and then to tear another sheet of scrip paper. He wrote me more prescriptions than would kill a baby elephant to shut me up. I was all of nineteen and not supposed to be wild and frantic? Not manic depressive.

The one thing I did know was, I was a recovering drug addict, and suffering. With years put in on the streets and running in flight or fight mode, I was beyond exhausted, felt lost, unprotected, and scared. Surrendering until my next battle was my stop here on a train of oblivion and being comatose.

When he spoke to me, his eyes were jet black and rolled whenever I had a suggestion about my care or change in medication. He was boss and I was a silly, young woman who did not know any better. Even though I knew my feelings, he knew them better, and what to over-medicate them with. Dr. Epstein was determined to keep me down and out no matter how many of the twenty medications he put me on.

More feelings—More dosage.

For a bit, I took it, being of ruined self and made of stone, I did not want to feel either way.

Only to shut down for a certain amount of time, the feelings as well as I began to rise. All bets were off and so was my insanity and ongoing panic attacks.

The flashes were maintaining their hold on me and I could not keep still and began to get myself mentally prepared for the war in my head and battle in my heart. I would have to be in for the long haul and change my life. This was not going to be easy. It was going to be the hardest thing in my life.

The feeling of being so-called treated by Princeton Joseph was beginning to feel all wrong. Nothing about it was right. As my panic attacks, and periods of relapse grew worse, as if they ever could, I was now on psychological medication to add to the self-destruction and self-hatred as well as cluelessness as to what was happening to my body, mind, and soul. The internal rumbling was growing louder and louder as my medications that could kill a baby elephant could not hold them at bay anymore.

Now, I began to fight, my final relapse, my tired rested strength welled up inside me as if I had no control or cared where I was about to go. Further than before and the mystery of the unknowns abounds me, this was no holds barred, and I was all in for the ride.

Once I made the decision to stay sober, synchronicity had taken its hold which I was as hell bent to move forward, and off the psychiatric medications.

Firstly, I lay in bed and detoxed myself from all of the medications that had held me back from my reality, no matter how horrible I could have imagined it. I was to keep going with every inch of power in my tiny cells of being. The sweats came, then the hallucinations took hold, I weathered through the darkest, most nightmarish of times.

Barely able to sit up after two weeks of crisis and withdraw, I started making the meetings again and talking to my acquaintances. One person gave me a name of her therapist, Patricia.

This time it felt right, the right place, at the right time. Painfully, I kept showing up to meetings and good things began to happen. Kerry gave me Patricia's number and the next day I got out of the coffin-bed. Still sweating and encompassed by the feeling of death, I prayed to God before my call, and I would find help.

I was desperate.

My shaky hand picked up the telephone and began dialing the numbers Kerry had written down on a ripped piece of paper that I mysteriously did not lose.

On the first ring Patricia answered, "Hello, this is Patricia, how can I help you?"

Going right in with a whispering voice, I raced, "Patricia, this is Dianne; Kerry gave me your number."

She already knew and said, "Yes, Dianne, I have been expecting your call. And I am very happy that you did so."

I asked, "You have?"

She responded, "Yes. So tell me, what has been going on?"

Ready as I ever was, I told her the truth, "I have been seeing Dr. Joseph and he prescribes me medication after medication to keep me down. It sounds weird, but I think he thinks I am neurotic and ridiculous every time I bring up memories or flashes." Abruptly I stopped and asked Patricia, "Please tell me I am at a loss, what should I do when these memories are haunting me?" Pausing and regaining my composer after yet another flash, I hammered her with more questions by asking her, "Patricia what does this mean when I have a vision of the past, should I remember it, what will happen? What is it? What does it mean?"

But Patricia, missing nothing, calmly stated, "Well honey, it is in my experience, if the flashes are coming, the brain is ready to tell you something, no matter what it is."

Finally, for the first time, in forever, I felt at ease.

She continued, "When is the next time you see Doctor Goldstein?"

"Later this week, at 10am," I told her.

Patricia suggested, "Well why don't we do this. At your next session with him, I will call you at his office, so while you are sitting there, we can explain what is going on with you." She continued with reassurance, "We can both talk to him and I can find out if he and I can work together and help you."

In agreement, I said, "Okay, and thank you, Patricia."

She ended the call with, "I will call at 10am this week, when you are at Dr. Goldstein's office and then we will set up an appointment afterward, so you and I can begin to talk."

Her voice stayed calm and assertive, while checking in with me one last time, "Dianne, how does that sound?"

"It sounds great. And I am looking forward to getting started with you and you talking to Dr. Joseph," I responded to her act of kindness.

She said, "All right. We'll all talk then."

"Thank you Patricia. Goodbye."

"Dianne, take care and be safe," she said.

Not wanting to leave her side, or her phone voice, I knew I had to move forward in my own way until we spoke again.

The rest of the week, I persevered and waited for my appointment with Princeton Joseph.

It came—the day—the time—the appointment. As soon as I walked into the doctor's office, I mentioned it to him that Patricia was calling at the beginning of the session.

Looking shocked, he reached for his scrip pad.

Nevertheless, before he could shell out another prescription I said, "I stopped taking everything about three weeks ago."

There was no need to explain, he tried to babble and make sense of it all. However, the phone rang into his office; it was Patricia, like clockwork.

Now he again was sweating, profusely. He reached for the phone as I could hear Patricia's sweet but stern voice, introducing herself to him. I could hear her on the other end of the phone.

He said a quick, "Hello."

Patricia maintained her composer as he was beyond short to her.

She introduced herself and explained her non-combative side of the situation, "Hi Doctor Goldstein. This is Patricia Randall. Dianne called me and has been experiencing flashbacks for a long- time now and would like to address them." Including him, she went on to say,

"I was hoping with your help we can help Dianne to work through these issues."

I could sense a small eye roll, but in contempt, he responded with more of a non-response, and said, "Well I don't think they are flashbacks. They are just a symptom of her mental illness."

Hearing the tone of her voice change, she alerted him, "I have been doing this for years, as you yourself have been too." He tried to cut her off and down, but she was not having it. Patricia stood her sacred ground, all in the name of saving me and doing me justice. She continued, "I believe when this happens it is time to explore the flashes that she is having and not ignore what her brain is trying to tell her."

Dr. Princeton abruptly said, "It is my educated guess that Dianne is making this up for attention." Moreover, shut her down.

Patricia must have realized she would get nowhere with him. As if, I ever could. She ended the call with him saying goodbye and asked if she could speak to me directly.

Another eye roll ensued as he handed me the phone.

I said meekly, "Hello, Patricia."

"Hi Dianne. How does next week, Monday at noon sound?"

I said, "Perfect."

I handed the phone back to Doctor Freud and without saying goodbye to Patricia, hung up the phone.

He tilted his head back into his pile of prescription pads and began to write more prescriptions He acted as if the last five minutes never even happened.

All he said was, "I am going to now prescribe y—"

Before he could finish, I headed for the door and said, "No thank you, I think you've done enough."

Prideful I walked out the door and into a new way of life.

4th Therapist
The One and Only

It was time. I knew it. I felt it. The right therapist—finally.

Patricia Randall was a well-educated therapist with many degrees from Cambridge and the right Boston universities. Although she did not just look great on paper, Patricia was a compassionate human being and refused to take a dime from me. Patricia said she would work out a sliding scale payment plan. She took nothing from me, and established an individual helpful mindset for every one of her clients.

Present time being 1990 and a big chunk of her name and the amazing frontier and pioneering practitioners accused of everything by the false memory institution. In addition, they were a no-good institution that would discredit anyone you tried to help survivors and call everyone crazy. They were wrong, I for one, knew I was getting better. For the first time in my life, I felt safe, sane, and sober. Patricia, NEVER ONCE, put an idea in my head or led me on some sort of chase. All she did was believe me until I could stand on my own two feet and even after I could stand on my own she still supported me.

There was one instance where the pressure in my head, (usually before a memory), became too great and I had a water bottle placed on her wicker coffee table. She always sat in the white, wicker rocking chair and I across from her in the wicker love seat. Another chair was in the room, but it was just there, for me, to stare at, I guess. This time no sooner did I sit down then I threw my water bottle from the coffee table across the room until it smashed into the wall across from us.

First, I held my head, yelling, "I can't, I can't take it anymore!"

Knowing this was serious, as it always was so intense with me; Patricia leaned into her coffee table and closer to me and asked, "What is too much for you Dianne?" In addition, asked, "What is going on?"

Literally, I lifted my body out of my chair and began blaming everything, around me, even myself. That all of this was garbage and then the rage took hold.

Suddenly, Patricia placed all of her four foot eleven inch frame between the door and me.

All the while, I was thinking, *is she crazy, I could kill her.*

I believe she knew this to be true as well, but nothing would stop her as she stood her ground.

Then, she repeatedly said, "Dianne, none of this is your fault. Dianne, none of this is your fault."

Shocked, I backed up, slowed down my thoughts and had the most vital memory of my little sister passing away at the hands of someone I loved the most.

I told her.

Tears welled up in her eyes as did mine. Then like a faucet the tears poured down my cheeks, ran off my chin, and onto the floor. Backing myself away from Patricia, I sat on the office windowsill with my legs curled up in front of me. Of course, Patricia standing beside me. Not to close, as she always knew, but close enough to let me know she was there for me.

She spoke softly and carefully, "Dianne, you are not to blame; you were six-years-old and could do nothing."

Agreeing with her, but still not sure, I believed to this day, I could have prevented my little sister's death. I did not. I fought for everyone's justice, including her, and it brought me to my knees every time.

Patricia, each time, caught me as I fell to my knees, with understanding she took it upon herself to be there for me every step of the way.

Since that time, our sessions, for a few years were from two to three intensive sessions a week. Still never charging me a dime. I began to see a future as I never could have before. Always believing in my heart that I would, and wanted to, be dead by the time I was twenty-one. In fact, at one time, this became my internal monologue and mantra for my life.

Because of Patricia Randall I began to see the light at the end of the tunnel. Just as if she said someday I would see it as well. Nevertheless, she had to see it first and for a long, long time before I even had a glimmer of light inside that extremely long tunnel of hopelessness and darkness.

She was and always will be the best therapist that ever happened to me. When I gave her credit for anything, she directed the credit back to me and said, "You did the work. I just help guide you."

As time when on, our sessions remained a steady once a week for a long period.

Thinking now, if I made it through those walls of hell, I could make it through college.

During our time together after eight years, I went to three colleges, attaining degrees and became an established member of society. Still kept my authentic self, as Patricia would have constantly put it when asking her a question, Patricia would say, "Be true to yourself."

Gradually, we went to phone sessions. Then every other week. Even through Patricia retired years before; she always held a session for me. Whenever I needed to talk.

After about fifteen years, Patricia, was sick, her lungs, her body, the stress of always helping others. This most loving, incredible, dynamic woman, I knew—became ill.

While on our last phone call, Charles, her husband was there, letting me know, the time had to be brief because she was on her deathbed.

Agreed.

Still Patricia focused on me saying, while struggling to breathe, "How are you doing honey?"

With urgency I asked, "Patricia, how am I going to make it? Then added, "I don't know how to move forward without you, and I feel like I still am not finished, there is more…"

I addressed her as if she was my mother dying and I did not know what to do next or how I was going to make it without her, or even what to do next.

Calmly and with ease Patricia said, "Dianne, you have been through hell and back, now it is time for you to live. You must move on and live. I promise you—it's time."

She gasped for what I could only imagine as her final breaths of air.

Charlie, lightly took the phone out of her hand and said, "Dianne, if you ever need anything please call me." In addition, continued, "Right now, Patricia and I are going to spend some time alone."

This was the last time I spoke to either of them. I knew Patricia, as strong as she was now in her seventies and was not going to make it. As frightened, lost, bewildered that I was, I took her direction, as I always have, and moved forward.

Still, I hear her tidbits of knowledge that will never leave me as she was a—only—mother to me.

Freely giving of herself with unconditional love and asking nothing in return.

I love you, Patricia.

5th Therapist
Dr. Frankenstein

Upon entering Cape Cod Psychiatric Unit. They put me on immediate protocol. Meaning I was going to meet with a psychiatrist and social worker every day. Therefore, my stay ensues.

In less than twenty-four hours, I met Dr. Frankenstein and my social worker, Jane, who would later become my next therapist. Jane first met me and we sat down. She told me the rundown of how protocol would work with Dr. Frankenstein.

Jane said, "Dianne, I think you are going to like Dr. Kemp. He is a really smart doctor."

Raising an eyebrow if I could in my state-of-mind, I replied, "That would be good."

Jane went over a couple of basic questions, the biological parents. These questions always got to me because it is and was too complicated to answer. I kept it short with "Yes" or "No" answers.

As we completed the questionnaire, Dr. Frankenstein walked into the room, the speed of his gait enticed me by his unkempt hair and messy appearance.

He sat down at his seat, next to Jane, and greeted me, "Well, hello Dianne, I am Doctor Kemp, and I will be treating and prescribing you the medications you'll need." He continued, "I am here only for six months and I am going back to Boston afterward, but I find that your story is quite different, in my file, please tell me more about yourself and your symptoms."

I began, stammering at first, "I… I was first diagnosed as manic depressive with Schizoid Effective Disorder at nineteen by another hospital, in Eagleville, Pennsylvania." I looked for a reaction, but the two of them just peered back at me, as if I was talking about gardening. So, I continued, "At the time, I was feeling like I was crawling out of my skin and I was also in acute detox from drugs, alcohol, and living on the streets of New York City—"

Doctor Frankenstein politely interrupted me to gather more information, and asked, "Are you sober now?"

Quickly, I answered, "Yes I am, and have been for over twenty years."

He was now successfully raising his one eyebrow and said, "Good for you, Dianne."

In agreement, Jane chimed in, "Excellent and impressive."

I continued, "Well, it has not been easy, I have been off my medications since nineteen years old and for the last twenty years the occasional doctor would prescribe me an antidepressant, which made my mind manic, to say the least."

"An antidepressant would make a manic-depressive person go out of control and completely manic," Dr. Frankenstein added.

"That is a bit of information I didn't know. Thank you for telling me." I looked up and they were both listening with the intent to help me and with great concern. Once again, I had the floor, I continued, "This is why I moved to the Cape. I had a feeling that I would get better here because in Philadelphia, where I had been a successful painter and professor, the cracks in me were becoming, craters and I was becoming more than unhinged. I knew that I was going to lose it. And time was running out."

Jane asked, "So, you moved here?"

My answer, "Exactly." Adding on, "Not knowing a soul."

She said, "Dianne, that took courage, to step into a place you never been and now you're here. You should be proud of yourself for getting help."

"Well, I had no more choice and I surrendered to the fact of my diagnosis, something I didn't do over twenty years ago." Looking up at both Dr. Frankenstein and Jane, I sincerely said, "I hit bottom with it, my illness only has gotten worse, a lot worse and untreated this time, I would have tried to commit suicide. The mania and depression were so bad, when manic; I would walk twenty-three hours a day, when depressed; I would paint non-stop and lie in bed the rest of the time in total darkness to desensitize myself." I stopped there, because now I felt listened to and gave them all the up-to-date information I had at this time.

Now, I waited for their reaction.

Never feeling ganged up on. Only feeling teamwork was ahead of me.

Doctor Frankenstein took the lead, "Again, Dianne, you have some story, and I believe we can help you, because you sincerely want to get better. I believe your first diagnosis was, and still is, right. I will prescribe your medicine, there are three, Depakote, this will stabilize your moods, Thorazine, and this is an antipsychotic, and lastly Lorazepam at bedtime to help you sleep through the night. You need to rest now, while you are in here, from not sleeping through your manic phase previously." He continued, "Jane and I will check in every day to see how well you are adjusting to the medication."

Jane nodded her head in agreement with Dr. Frankenstein.

I was grateful for them. The power of the two of them, I believe they would help me.

Simply, I said, "Sounds good."

He said, "Great, we will get you started on your medications immediately and if you need anything, anything at all please go to the nurse's station to your assigned nurse and she will get in touch with us. If we do not hear from you, we will see you tomorrow, approximately the same time."

Feeling secure, I stood up from my chair, not wanting to leave my security blanket, and went back out into the psychiatric unit.

During my stay at Cape Psych Center, I worked with Dr. Frankenstein and Jane every day for several days. Jane would secure me, by letting me know that she would be my therapist once a week on the outside. Doctor Frankenstein was going to keep in touch with me by calling me in a week to continue to see how I was adjusting outside of the unit and back into real life on the medication regime.

In fact, before I left the unit, I felt much better on this dosage and these medications then I have ever felt. Not in a manic-way but in a very real-way. My feet were on the ground and they were ready to walk out of the unit and into life with the help of Jane's guidance as my next therapist.

6th Therapist
On the Outside with Jane

By the time I walked into her office, outside the hospital, Jane was ready, with a not so generic pad of papers, a file on me, and above all a look of concerned look of happiness. Because I reached her, on time, and took my seat ready for battle within my internal self.

She took a deep breath and so did I.

Jane started with an important question, "Dianne how was the first week outside the hospital for you?"

Honestly, I answered, "Well… It has been calmer, I had been calmer, and knowing that I was going to see you for therapy helped a lot." Then I had to tell her, "You see my therapist back in New York, Patricia, guided me for years, and she passed away when I was living in Philadelphia that is when the cracks became sinkholes." As I was in some sort of race against time, I kept going, "Patricia helped me, with memories, life, growing up." Then I added, the ultimate truth, "You remind me of her."

I did not expect you to be her but her presence was comforting to me. I trusted her.

Jane welcomed my insight and had a smile on her face as she said, "Dianne, I am glad that I remind you of such a pivotal person in your life." She shifted in her seat and the tone in her voice became for serious when adding, "I am her to guide, help, and support you through anything and everything. These sessions are about you, how you are feeling and navigating through life."

Even though Jane was good for me, I knew there was a part of me that she would not reach, which Patricia did, my whole self, memories and all. I felt as if I could touch on them and talk about some memories, but I had to focus on thr present moment and growing. Jane along with meetings would get me through this foreseen rough patch.

The first session we were very compatible among each other. She was open with me as I was with her. We communicated with simplicity and as well as complexity's hardships in my life.

She was most fascinated about me being from a homeless adolescent background and moving into a full scholarship educated young person, growing up to become a successful, sensitive, and truthful oil painter. Then above all an established professor in and around Ivy League Universities to teaching other medical professors ten times older than myself all the way to individual artist's that could not afford classes. All the while maintaining my professional business, a good name with integrity, and financial success. But I let her know, this all came at a steep price, no family, small circle of friends, only business individuals who I can trust, because when you reach that level of success, everyone wants something, including what I valued most—my privacy. Interviews and exhibitions pushed me to the limit. I was not a people-person and the galleries and museums I exhibited at knew I had a reputation for not showing up at my own exhibitions. They learned to put it in my contract to show, down to the hours I have to be there during my exhibit, I had to sign on the dotted line. Only on certain dates was the person who commissioned my work allowed in the studio. Models had to sign paperwork stating no looking at work contracts. They were not good about this, they would not return.

My temperament was that of an insanely private painter. There were gallerists haunting me in the city at my recovery meetings. I had solid recovery and protected it like a fierce mama loin protecting her offspring. By the end of Philadelphia, the paranoia and isolation only grew deeper. The only way to dig myself out was to plan for a year, pack paintings, office, and studio. Hire movers and move once all my contracts fulfilled. I was not running from something; I was running to something. Cape Cod, a new life, more peaceful, and private.

I told Jane, "Immediately, I started going to meetings, took a coffee commitment, because I am so shy, got a sponsor, and kept through the steps—again."

We stayed an extra half an hour after session to complete my, "Life's Story."

I apologized, "Jane I am so sorry, I went on and on. Thank you for listening."

Jane said, "No, Dianne this is all so important, because it got you where you are today. Sitting here in my office." She continued, "Stress is a huge factor for you and getting triggered by your isolation." She resumed, "The most important issue is for me is to learn as much as I can about you. I think you are amazing, to have gotten to where you are, not were, but are, accepting yourself."

My response to her was, "I simply pulled myself out of the dumps, no matter what the costs, and decided to try to live again."

"Well, it takes great courage, to walk away from it all; to get help for your mental, emotional, and physical health," she said.

I replied, "Thank you, but the choice was life or death. It seems to always come down to that for me." Perplexed I said, "I don't know why but I chose life. Even though, I know what is out there and have seen the worst, I continue to trust God's process."

Jane comforted me by saying, "You deserve the best and I will make sure you get the best care."

I shook my head, cupped my hands, and gently placed my embarrassed red face that was flooded with tears.

Not being able to speak, my face feeling flushed, with a rush heat.

Jane spoke for a moment, "There is no need to ever feel embarrassed by sorrow, you are allowed to feel, you are entitled to feel, Dianne."

She had a kindness, as Patricia had, and a generosity for my well-being, to feel that someone who was invested in my recovery made me feel safe, secure, and proud. I believe my self-esteem that day went up twenty points—going from no self-esteem to low self-esteem.

Jane and I continued to have sessions for over a year and a half. Throughout these sessions, I revealed so much about my past, different parts, behaviors, and patterns. With her help, I was able to continue to stay on the straight and narrow.

Then she revealed to me that she was retiring, because her husband was retired now and he wanted to spend more time with her, but she would continue to see me and only a couple of other clients. I think *behind her husband's back*. Still once a week and going strong.

Our time together was precious to me. It was a confessional as well as a memory bank. What I liked about Jane was that she not only had a sense of humor, but she got it. Truly, she was on my side and helped me navigate very carefully through the world by keeping emotionally healthy and mentally aware in life. The outside world and people, I still after forty years did not trust, but at this age, I accepted my illness and myself. Nevertheless, the terror may never end. I had my own paranoia but put at ease every time with Jane. I trusted no one in life and in many directions from anyone who was able to break through my steel walls.

Jane did tell me; eventually she would retire permanently the more her husband pushed. In my opinion, I believed she loved what she did; helping the sick and suffering, and her compassionate nature was never lost on me.

The one subject matter that she or I did not shy away from was my biological father. He tricked me every day, I believed him, and that the night-father was different from the day-father. Although the daytime dad beat the crap out of me, broke my nose several times, before I was four years old. The never-ending crying, tears, emotions, and feelings came down on both of us hard. The molestation alone would be enough for her. I did not get into the major abuse that surrounded me like Fort Knox in my childhood. However, Jane was able to take on a lot. Patricia received the brunt of my anger and rage, helping me move forward to anyone else with them being less scared. Jane was compassionate, but I knew she did not have Patricia's bravery.

Then it came, almost out of nowhere, Jane announced, "Well Dianne, I have to retire."

Now, I cried.

She continued, "I am sorry, my husband now has demanded that I retire, from *all* clients, and I gave notice at Cape Cod Healthcare Hospital too. It was a big decision for me, and if it were up to me, I would still see you. Nevertheless, I promised him, and he wants us to see the world and travel. We are both seventy and as you know he retired a couple years back, and now I have been seeing you for well over a year now."

I just kept crying.

Jane explained further, "I thank you for the last couple of years, and to tell you the truth, as always, you are the one client, I am seeing up until the last minute. I know you benefit from our sessions so much and I also know how grateful you are, so I will give you my number and call me if you would like to meet for lunch, just to talk, it is up to you. But I have to do this—"

Through my tears, I had to tell her how I felt, "Jane, I am scared, worried, of course, about myself. I knew this was coming, you told me…"

I just could not hold back the tears and now the air was dissipating around me. I could hardly inhale.

Jane saw the struggle and tried to ease me, "Dianne, I will be with you, in your transition, and I will make sure you get set up with the right therapist."

Somewhat it helped as I felt more at ease, I tried not to make her feel guilty, and I had no idea I would react this way.

Now, a hot mess, Jane handed me the tissue box on the end table, and I pulled a few out, managing to wipe my face down and wring it out, I let out a deep sigh, while looking at her a whole heartily said, "Thank you, Jane, for everything you helped me with."

Graciously Jane said, "You're welcome." Like Patricia reminded me, "You showed up every week and did the work." Then she changed her tone into a question-like demand, "Dianne, promise me you will keep up the good work and work hard with the new therapist."

I answered, "Okay, I promise." With a follow up question, then I asked her, "Who do you have in mind for me?"

Without hesitation she stated, "Her name is Jennifer, and she is good and also part of the Cape Cod Healthcare Center, she has openings in the next two weeks, so we can still complete our sessions until then."

Now, I hesitated and wanted to ask her more about Jennifer, but I would rather wait and see my first impression of her and continue the session with Jane about the loss of yet someone else I trusted.

Needless to explain that I was playing the victim at that session. I wanted to be comforted.

Jane was motherly, as she too knew that is always what I needed. We spoke less about my mother in all sessions, which became clearer to me later.

It was clear to me that Jane had the gift of kindness. Being at the right place at the right hospital, at the right time, was a gift from a power great than myself.

She was for me by a power greater than I was. I would be forever be grateful for her kinship and kindness.

7th Therapist
The Breather

Our session started normal and I liked Jennifer. I thought Jane did a good job in picking my next therapist. Jennifer Traitor. She was part of the Cape Cod Healthcare Network and she told me that Jane spoke highly about me. My beige file was on her desk, I glanced down at it, and saw words in circled caps, "ABOVE AVERAGE INTELLIGENCE." Not knowing if that was a "Proceeding with caution." It reminded me of my first cat, Rembrandt, and his folder said, "CAT WILL BITE, PROCEED WITH CAUTION," with a sticker of a mouth of fangs having the same circle around them. Unsure, if *I* should have proceeded with caution.

Jennifer kept the file opened, as it was obvious my glance was more like a stare. She was open and wanted me to be the same with her. There was something about Jennifer, this one; I could not put my finger on right away.

Then it came. As she pulled up her sleeves to get down to working with me. I noticed her tattoo on her delicate wrists. She rolled rough and tough but when it came to her ankle and wrists Jennifer was displaying bird bones. She did not let my glance of shock pass.

Jennifer looked at her tattooed wrist and then looked at me with a direct stare and wanting me to know, as if she was in therapy, she asked, "Are you looking at the tattoo on my wrist, Dianne, and wondering who it is?"

I didn't dare to ask, but I did anyway, "Yes. Why do you have a tattoo? Adding, "It doesn't seem right?"

She came back with a response, "Well, since you asked, it is very private to me, Donnie, *was* my son and he died last year."

While explaining to me the meaning of her tattoo, she came closer and showed me it, so I could see it up close and personal.

She wanted a reaction from me and could see she was getting one. The sadness inside me was welling up to the form of uncontrollable tears because I felt sad for her, and for her son. In addition, I felt his death was untimely in the form of a drug overdose.

I paused from my feeling.

Jennifer took to my feeling and then asked me, "How does that make you feel, Dianne?"

Not withholding as the tears, I was trying to hold back, I could feel her pain, his pain, and my pain for them. Unexpectedly the feelings of deep sorrow compounded inside of me.

I said, "I feel sad. This is sad." Knowing the answer and seeing her face of confused sorrow, I asked anyway, "How did Donnie pass away."

She was straightforward in her answer and said, "He was only nineteen and died of a drug overdose."

Responding to her tone of loss and guilt in her voice, I was still curious, I implied, "Heroin?"

She said, "Yes. That and opiates." Then she explained, "He would get sober, then pick up, it was a roller coaster ride for years. He had a year and a half, then picked up, and died instantly."

I knew that the session had shifted onto Jennifer, but I felt like she was swimming in a deep rip current unable to leave this not-so-distant memory behind. She carried it with her, like her cross to bear."

She checked in with me, "Dianne, are you feeling."

"It is all too sad. Too soon. For both of you. And I am sorry for your incredible loss, Jennifer."

Reaching for my hand and holding it, she drew her head down and said a heartfelt, "Thank you."

Jennifer had a way of being open about herself; in turn, it helped me feel less judged, as she knew what it took for this reformed, sober woman, who had struggled. The struggle of getting and staying sober never ended and I let her know it.

"Jennifer, even after all this time; there are times in my life when the struggle of keeping my sobriety is all too hard. I hang on for my dear life and I was told, this too shall pass. I keep recovery first, but lately, I have been isolating more, hating the program, and the principle over personalities is not working for me."

The noticeable resentment towards the program was obvious, she spoke at the program and its people by responding, Jennifer agreed, "I hate the program. They are a bunch of sick losers and they never get better, only temporarily."

My heart sank, because all the therapists I had worked with up until this point always were-in agreement with the program.

Secretly I was glad. This almost gave me permission to drink.

I came clean with Jennifer and agreed with her.

Even though it felt wrong, I said, "Yes. You are right. I am glad someone sees it for the way I do. As a matter of fact, I have been planning to have a cocktail in the next six months."

Sick of holding the secret, I was glad to have let it go.

Jennifer complied, which I knew, was not good.

We still met every week and grew closer. I told her my secrets and my eccentric ways and she liked that I was different. Dealing with a lot of emotions and present moment happenings.

The sessions seemed to grow more surface by the week.

After she came back from a seminar, something bizarre happened... Jennifer learned a new technique. However, it was not so new to the rest of the western hemisphere. She called it breathing. On the other hand, hyperventilating.

Now every time it became too intense or difficult for her or for me to process, or so she thought, she resorted to throwing her arms wide and said, "Okay, Okay, let's do the breathing technique I showed you, in for three, hold, out for three." She would encourage me. "Come on, big deep breath in, hold—"

Her face now purple and dramatic gestures, I was embarrassed not just for myself but her too.

She continued, as I followed her guidance. And deep breath out." With a huge blow out, like when a tire blows out on the roadway. She blew out as my hair flew back from the breeze.

I pretended just to go along. Nevertheless, I knew this could be the end. Not being truthful was the worst thing that could happen. That is exactly what was happening. I thought this was a stupid exercise and her dramatics only made me feel embarrassed for the both of us—I recoiled.

Knowing my days were numbered, being sober after twenty-six years began, for the first time to lose its luster. I could not see myself with Jennifer anymore.

Now I wanted to use, and I wanted to stop breathing at the end of each session. Or have her stop me in the middle of something I needed to feel and have me breathe like a psychotic ameba having an aneurism.

This would hurt her, but I told her I was going to cut down on our sessions and try to get through on my own issues. Two sessions left to one.

Then none.

8th Therapist
The Well not

Michelle was not in the network of my insurance so rather she would be paid with one of my paintings. Before she saw me, she researched me, Dianne Corbeau the painter. Although this was beneficial to me, my work history entered the door before I did and followed me to a predestined fate with her.

I talked a lot about painting, how much I have been painting, but for the first time since I was sixteen, or in my life, I had lost interest in painting.

Even through depressions, I would paint, nonstop. By now, this feeling of listlessness was different. Uninterested and bored with not having a person to paint or draw and only seascapes and repetitive landscapes, it could not hold my interest anymore. This was worse than depression. This was the undesired willingness to show up at the easel every morning and I could not accept the mediocrity on the Cape anymore so figured I might as well quit. Which meant, quit everything, including sobriety, and anything else that was doing the next right thing. Meetings all fell by the wayside as I found myself drinking again. It was never social. I tried with friends, but from the first day on. I was at the liquor store by 8am every day, and then made sure I had enough whiskey and wine to last me, throughout the night. As I needed to have it every fifteen minutes or seizures would ensue. This while my esophagus began to swell and bleed, cutting my air pipe off and my eyes swollen shut. Rapidly over two years of relapse after twenty-six years of sobriety was horrendous pain, not only mentally but emotionally, and physically (breaking my leg in eight places and getting no help because it would come between me and my drinking).

I saw Michelle for the first year's sessions, they were easy and I would just go in so I would have someone to talk to. She did not know I was drinking, even though the smell of booze was coming out of my pores.

Then she asked for a painting. I asked her if this was the end of therapy. Michelle said no but now I needed to start paying her on a sliding scale because she still wanted to see me.

We agreed. I kept my word, as she wanted a seascape, which was good for me.

The next session I brought her about five seascapes, all framed from previous exhibitions. She picked the one with the flock of birds flying over the crashing sea of waves. I was happy she picked that one.

The drinking began to catch up with me. During this time, I managed to keep my head afloat in the darkest hours. Literally, my reaction to alcohol was allergic. Apparently, if I had any questions going into this relapse if I was an alcoholic, I would have the answered—clearly—yes.

During this time, I met a platonic friend, Alexander, he would drive me places, as therapy, and I began to get honest with Michelle. It was the least I could do. After leaving her for a few months to make more time for my drinking, I returned to her. Alexander came into my session with her so it would be easier for me to tell her what I had been doing for the last few months. I told Michelle he would be there and when we walked into her office, there were three chairs nothing in between us. We were all out in the open.

Walking into her office I felt like I was walking over hot coals and Alexander gave me the strength to take one more step into the chair. Michelle took one look at me and knew; I was so far gone that I needed to go somewhere.

On the ride there, I was still forcing down alcohol all night, and morning. As I poured it down my rock-solid swollen gullet it came immediately right back up. In Alex's car, out the window, and so on. The trick was sipping until my mouth would stop bleeding and the vomits would go away.

I was not going to live. This was my constant thought. Furthermore, I was not going to live if I kept drinking, but the fear of withdrawal was killing me. Because I knew, if I went somewhere and withdrew from the alcohol there was over a 90% chance I would die.

In Michelle's office, I revealed to her the truth. With Alex, being there made it more real. I lost my license as well; to do with drinking, of course. I believed I hit bottom. This was the worst.

They recommended that I go to Cape Cod Hospital and commit myself, to which I agreed. I did not feel ganged up on, we were all in agreement. This was a must and the last thing I could do.

It meant a lot to me that Michelle did not hold resentment but admitted that this was way out of her league and that I needed professional help. I needed to be behind brick walls and unable to walk out of the place to get to a liquor store.

As the session was a full sixty minutes, it flew by, knowing my fate was now to fess up and go to the Emergency Room. Trying to keep me on the Cape would be no small feat. It was summer and I am sure the beds filled and they would ship me of to another mental ward, because they did not take in dual diagnosed patients.

When we were done, leaving Michelle's office, Alexander and I knew our next step. We took it and that was the last time I spoke with Michelle.

9th Therapist
The Hawaii Hit On

Fresh out of the hospital and landing into the "New" therapist's lap. Vulnerable, unbelievable and shaken to my core. I showed up on Hawaii Five O's doorstep, like a wet puppy dog, needing help, compassion, and leadership, to keep me away from a drink.

No sooner did I get there than Hawaii's began to give me her pitch. First session, she did not waste one minute.

Eileen was her name and nailing me was her game.

She was sitting at her wide-angle twenty-five inch monitor computer and admittedly in a proud like manner said, "I must confess Dianne, I looked you up on search engines and your name proceeds you."

My luck, someone who thinks she idealizes me, does not even think about the real, messed up me.

Being only a week out of the hospital, I was sober now for three weeks. She was my assigned therapist on Cape Cod to continue my aftercare. I have no gay radar and if someone hit on me it would go right over my head. Especially, right now.

She gushed about my achievements and I waited patiently until I could begin. It looked like that was not going to happen… Then it happened.

Eileen asked, "So I think you are amazing, but enough about that, how was your transition getting out of the hospital and into the stream of life?"

Finally, I began, "Well," with an eye roll, "It has been one hell of a week. I continued quickly so she could not cut me off, "Eileen, this has been the worst week of my life. I am struggling, with every minute of every day. I have to focus on getting well."

No sooner did I pause, again tearful.

She cuts me off, as if I said nothing and became like every other person in my world of not seeing exactly what I was telling you.

I was saying to her, I was dying, she was hearing, I must go teach at your frigid rich people day camp in Hawaii and be a lead professor for you, to make you look good.

In all honesty, I did not ever know if I could or would be sober by June of that year. It was a long time away and I vowed never to teach again, once I left the city, and moved to the Cape a couple of years ago.

Her knee was shaking like an impatient child trying to get my attention. Loud and clear.

I gave her the floor, as I gave up without even trying,

She went on, now pulling her chair next to me, and turning her monitor around.

Eileen started to state her case, "Look at you, you will be teaching, in Honolulu, Hawaii. She looked over at me for my reaction.

Instead, I gave her a deadpanned, "Okay."

You will be on vacation practically every day. You will get to design your own classes: Anatomy, figure, portrait painting, and landscape painting just to name a few. To have a professor of your caliber come and teach our students would be great. Now don't get me wrong, we have a waiting list for professional and famous professors that we would bump off the first spot and put you on there as the headliner." She came up for air, then went right back to admitting, "I know I shouldn't even propose this to a client, it is ethically wrong, and I can get fired for this. But I think it would be a great time and you need to get away and go on vacation."

I thought, *God, is this sale's pitch over with yet?*

She almost replied to my thought by asking, "So, what do you think, Dianne?"

My response, "Well, it all sounds good Eileen, but to tell you the truth, I don't know if I even want to teach again, and I really need to think about it. I mean I just got sober."

Then she did the worst thing possible, she gestured, the "Milton Mouth." A sneak is a sneak is a sneak. She was a dishonest sneak who not only wanted to bed me but make herself look good while doing it.

She replied, "Well take time to think about it. We have a few months to decide but I wanted to get you while I have you here."

Her self-satisfaction she let out her sales pitch exhale and now she was ready to continue the session.

Eileen said, "Please Dianne let's talk about you, your time, I am sorry, I got lost in the moment of excitement."

This of course confused me because it was now, which is when she was concerned for me. It must be part of her manipulation as there were ten minutes left and we spent the remainder of the time talking about my stay in this furious hospital that was all wrong. The abuse taken in the hospital, I was trying to tell her, I was damaged, broken, and at this point insane.

I was talking to a puppet of stammering shame of hiding who she really was. Offering this poor girl glitz and glamour, when all I really wanted was for the unshakable pain to fall off me.

The session was ending, and she could not help herself by saying, "So you'll think about it, Dianne, won't you?"

To people please I said, "Yes, I will think about it and let you know."

My concern was still therapy I was so desperate for help and confused as to what she did I asked, "When are we seeing each other again?"

Her immediate rebuttal was, "Yes, same time and place next week." Adding on, "If you want to keep your therapy appointments in the same time slots that is what we will do". Then a check in, "How does that sound, Dianne?"

"Sounds good to me, see you next week," I replied

Then something weird happened, as if this appointment was not weird enough. Eileen put her hand out and shook it. I found that odd. I felt wronged twice over. Now she wanted to shake my hand to seal-the-deal."

I returned her gesture and shook her hand. It felt like I was making a deal with the devil.

Opposing on going to the next session, I went out of curiosity. Still not drinking and knew that whatever little therapy I did get from her was almost worth it. I figured I would give it another try and told her, 'I do not want to teach,' and that was it. I spoke to my sponsor all week about it. Obsessing over this situation went from; I vowed to myself never teach again. It was a trigger for my anxiety right now. Anxiety was my way via the bottle.

The real answer, the only answer was, NO.

By the second session, I had more anxiety than the first. This was not the norm.

Walking into her office, she seemed calmer; maybe she saw the expression on my face upon entering.

With a deep sigh, she had to ask, not giving me the months of thought she said I could have.

She asked, "Dianne, I just wanted to ask, if you have given the teaching job in Hawaii any thought?" I thought, *shameless.*

Simply, I said, "Yes," followed with, "no."

She did get the point. I did not want to talk about it anymore. I wanted to get help. I was willing to give her another chance, out of desperation.

She followed me by just giving me a look of disappointment, then changed her facial expression to her game face, perked up in her chair, and said, "Okay. Okay. Not a big deal, it would have just been great to have you.

The rest of the second session was Eileen squirming in her chair and if I mentioned painting, she would circle back to Hawaii and asking questions such as, "Will you ever teach again?"

I knew this was a non-working therapist-client relationship. My desperation and confusion of her liking me grew into self-respect and new founded self-esteem. Learning how to say, "No," in-order to save my recovery. Because I knew from that point on, my recovery was more important than anything was and I began to trust my gut again. To me this was a sign to give this therapist up, not set another appointment, and move on.

When it was time to leave this time, Eileen nervously stood up and wanted the repetition from the last session. She motioned out her hand for a handshake and I held my hand tightly by my side.

Informing her, "This will be the last time, thank you."

She said, "Okay." Speechless (If you could imagine).

I turned away from her and walked swiftly out the door with my head held high.

10th Therapist
The Assigned Psychiatrist

Timothy was quite different from many other psychiatrists. He was very down to earth and humble as a psychiatrist could be. Even though we were on borrowed time, we were able to talk. I have gotten to know him as a real humanitarian. Using his talents and education to go to Sweden and teach people that were disabled, English. Timothy said, he took time "off," meaning he did not get paid." Because it showed to him when he worked with, them and they learned a new language that the part of the brain that is mentally ill, or "out-of-control." Gains for strength and control for the ups and downs in manic depressive patients as well as Aids patients in various mental illness states and helps to support and control the Limbic System through the same temporal lobe in the brain.

All this information I gathered from him, from a poster he hung on his wall of Sweden. I complemented the red fiery poster hanging under precious glass, as if it was his most prized possession.

Immediately, I liked Timothy. By taking notice of his room, all his diplomas, which I read on my way to being seated, from Yale to braille. He was with honors always graduating. He also hung them for himself to see, behind the patient. Almost to remind himself of where he came from. Now, he was not poor, he dressed well, almost too well to fit the bill as a psychiatrist. But he understood, the one thing that any psychiatrist ever did, or doctor for that matter, the degrees, so many that he earned were his, not to intimate the patient or a "See how smart I am," statement. He really wanted to understand you as an individual and your mind.

Timothy told me, "Dianne, it is what I love to do, help people who have these, if you will, disabilities of the mind."

I could tell that going to Sweden and having the poster was his way of giving back and loving what he does.

Explaining to him, "I auction off my paintings now to help charities, from the blind people to the animals."

He replied, "Well you have a lot to give, so don't give up on yourself."

My answer was almost an unbelievable, "Okay, I will keep trying. Life has gotten to me, I feel and am, broken. Once again, I blame myself, and hate myself. I am at the bottom rung."

Timothy loved to discuss the mind and every facet involved with it. That was fascinating to me. He, out of all the doctors, would be open enough and have knowledge to share with me the anatomy of the brain, its rebuilding, and working with mental illness.

He must have read in my beige folder that I studied neurology and anatomy of the brain in medical school as well as carried out my studies and observations years later, from squirrels, birds, turkeys, elephants, and human beings, with and without different illnesses both physical and mental.

Timothy found that fascinating, as we spent the rest of our first session, refills, not many prescriptions, but just enough to level out my manic depression.

My illness was hard to pin down, as it was based on stress episodes, seasonal, come to find out my environment.

Noticing my folder as he opened and closed it, I looked up nervously at him. He made light of it and said, "Yes. We are going to either tape this one together or get you another folder.

Timothy put through my non-narcotic refills to the pharmacy, through the computer, and then rescheduled me for one month he was a great new psychiatrist at Cape Cod Behavior Health and my first impression proved the people who told me this to be right.

It proved that he was not only well educated but, he cared. Which was rare.

I did not even know, if *I* cared enough—to live.

Being fresh out of the hospital, and being hit on by another therapist, I knew know at least I was guarded with a good head doctor.

From then on, Timothy adjusted my medications, always believed in me, and even if I got sent back to the hospital or the emergency room, and doctors thought I was "Drug seeking."

He knew I was not and would prescribe whatever medication I lost, dropped, or whatever brain damaged thing I would do. Even taking my medication like clockwork. Once in a while, I messed up, one time it fell in the toilet. I swear my heart dropped, but I learned not to keep my medications over the toilet, or sink, or even in the bathroom.

Continually, I reported to him, through Covid-19 and all sorts of changes through my life. He does not treat me like a mentally ill disabled female. However, a smart human being who can make mistakes and learn from them.

I have seen other doctors treating me, and getting angry at him, because he would go against them. I know he had fought for me. When other quacks took away medication and put me in solitary confinement, Timothy would help me on the outside.

He listens and responds, appropriately. Not your "normal psychiatrist."

I won when I did get fit with Timothy. This gave me the flicker of hope I needed to drop the "Hawaii Therapist." Now, I was ready, and had hope I would be able to find a new therapist, like Patricia to help me go further with my abuse issues, because now there was more was left, my memories were coming toward me like a runaway train, in the here and now.

I could not back away and begun my search.

11th Therapist
The Green Maureen

My search began. It was not easy.

Starting with Psychology Today, with Massachusetts therapists, anyone that would have on their resume specific training I would need as there were numerous internal issues and to clean up the old ones left from working with Patricia. Knowing it would not be easy, I would have horrible breakdowns along the way. My hopes would be up with someone, only for them to say, they do not take insurance, if they could, they would put me on a waiting list. I said to them, "Great." Knowing I would never hear from them again.

After four-months of messages and searching, a nice therapist called me from Cambridge, Massachusetts.

She spoke to me very kindly, and in an immediate tone said, "Hello, Dianne. This is Dr. Holbrook. You are not going to believe this, my practice is full, but I did a search for what you needed, and I have four names to give you that take your insurance and practice what you need and also are taking new clients."

I thought, *this couldn't be happening, "My guardian angel."*

Instead, I exclaimed, "Wow, this is unbelievable! Thank You!"

She went on to ask, "Do have a pen and paper ready? I could give you their information."

"Yes. I am all set. I've been for years,"

I was half joking but serious, grabbed the first piece of paper I saw, and pen that worked, hovered over the table, and confirmed to her, "I am ready, with paper and pen."

She gave me the names, numbers, and locations of all four therapists. Then she said, "Out of these four you should find one that works for you."

I told my guardian angel, "Yes. I will call them now and leave them messages."

She helped me even further by saying, "Dianne, once you call them, interview them, and see if they are a good fit for you. Also, if you cannot find someone, call me back, and we'll search further."

I said, "I cannot believe you called me with this information. I've been trying so hard and have found no one."

"Well, she replied. "You are welcome Dianne, it is the least I can do, I can feel your pain through the phone, and I have a feeling one of these therapists will be able to help you. If not, like I said, call me back, we might have to broaden our search off out of Massachusetts."

"Okay. And I will call you if nothing happens." Thank you again, Dr. Holbrook." I said with a calmer voice.

Knowing I was not alone in my quest to find a therapist helped me, tremendously.

No sooner did I hang up the phone, I had the therapists' names and numbers written down on a piece of paper.

It began, but a more faithful search.

I called all four therapists and within the week's end they called me back.

The first one I went to see, was not a good fit, not deep enough.

Second one, left a message on my machine, thought, Hawaii Five O again, would call her if others did not work.

Third was Joyce, sounded very genuine and nice, so I saw, her. I was going to pick her.

The fourth, Maureen, she was curious, knowledge about my circumstances of unfinished business, and more than anything determined to help me out of this hell hole. Most importantly, she was compassionate, and we connected. Our conversation flowed and she was easy to talk to.

I felt in that room, that I found my therapist/psychologist.

Maureen and I agreed to meet next week, same time, for my session. She had a friend who was a specialist on my issues, in California, who would help us through, and she would research even more books, to help me on all levels. She was green in certain departments, but knowledgeable in many others.

Feeling as if I was back in therapy again. For the first time in years, I felt many feelings, but most of all safe. Now, I could get started on getting better, with a great emotional recovery, sponsorship, and the program.

After our interview session, our next session, we both got down to work on my memories and emotions. Maureen did mention during our interview and our last session that she would be speaking to a specialist on this specific subject matter. Although she had some experience, she was humble enough to admit she needed more help to understand what was happening. Even though we started working, I could tell Maureen was a workhorse like me, and that she has already read in one week about a five-hundred-page book about the subject in one night.

Being impressed with her showing up and really taking me seriously. Many people, even therapists, would tell you that you are crazy, and I do not blame her, it does sound crazy. The perpetrators want it to sound crazy, and I should have lost my mind years ago.

I had one "best" friend before I moved to Cape Cod, Nora, used to tell me, "It is amazing you are not in a padded room, with what you have been through."

Nora did not know the half of it either.

Maureen felt the same way as there was constant back and forth flow to our conversions. She would be able to read me and look for signs. Nevertheless, I was able to read her as well. She was transparent and honest. One never finds those qualities anymore in people let alone therapists. Maureen comforted me that she knew the difference if I said, "O' my God I want to die to, "I am going to kill myself." I believed her and signed the paperwork only if she included both of us, if she feels like I was suicidal, that she was only alowed to contact Timothy, with me present and vice-versa.

It was the only way for me to sign. She we agreed and signed it.

We went through one session a week until we got to more than heavy issues and she pushed, literally, pushed my intense sessions to two times a week.

Maureen said, "It is because I really do care about you, Dianne. But if I get audited which every one of my colleagues, that I meet with once a week, is telling me I will then—"

"Maureen I will back you up in court, I really appreciate your faith in me. I said, gratefully."

She replied, "Well you will have to write a short note before each second session saying if you do not receive this extra session, then you will want to commit suicide, or something of the like."

"Agreed," I replied.

Maureen kicked up her sessions with her adviser, or therapist, on her own dime and continued, both worked intensely in her office with me. I had what she called "kick back." This usually happened on Friday's and I would have to write and draw in my trusty red, thousand-page art book. *Why the grids, why this book?* I do not know, but it helped me feel comforted.

Each therapy book helped me explain what was happening inside of me. It would slow me down enough for the memories to stop and the writing and drawing would produce the memories.

I did emotionally lose it from time to time. One time Maureen got off the phone with the specialist in California and said to me, "The way Patricia did things with you was fine back then. It was what they knew and what they did that helped you. She did nothing wrong. But now Dianne, there is a different way."

She described it to me, and it overwhelmed me and I lost it.

I called her on the phone, while walking as I usually did after our sessions, to process the most painful parts of me. Therefore, I left her a message, knowing she was still in the office.

Maureen phoned me right back, speaking to me calmly, she explained, what led to a to another emotional episode.

Then the weirdest event happened during my conversation with her, while I was out for a walk and on the phone with her.

A large coyote crossed my path, and walked over my feet, to get from the beach side to the marsh. He galloped really. Neither one of us paying any mind to one another.

Once he was across, and in the marsh, walking with me, almost beside me.

Acknowledged the coyote by telling Maureen as she was explaining, "Maureen you are not going to believe this, but a coyote just walked on my feet and is walking with me right now."

She only paused for a moment. Then continued to bring me back, and sounded stressed, "Dianne, this is very important that you understand this and not get too overwhelmed because it is going to take time."

My stunned response was, "What?" and "Okay." I was willing to go deeper and have the pain stop. I felt that this was the first time I was getting the continued help that I needed that Patricia and me could not finish up.

She also ended the conversation with a compliment. "Even the specialist said you were smart or really believed in spirituality. She has never seen someone in her office go through these issues so fast." Then Maureen comforted me, "Dianne, it will be okay. We are in this together. I am not going to leave you and I have gotten us the extra help we needed. You are an intelligent person who is quite emotional, as anyone who had been in your shoes would be." As if I would ever interrupt a compliment. She continued, "So we are going to work on this and now I will be checking in with the specialist, twice a week, since we are meeting more." Adding on, "I am doing this because I believe in you."

I was leery because I was stepping once again into the unknown, but I had nothing to lose and everything to gain. This was a lot of work already, the intensive crying, real core pain, anger, rage, and "sheet therapy" as my sponsor named it.

Even if Maureen betrayed me, I thought, at least I would get as well as I could. I always felt against the clock with these embedded issues. I did not know if it was going to end. "So," I told Maureen, "Thank you for helping me and returning my call as quickly as you did, I appreciate all the work and faith you are having with me. It makes me want to work even harder." Adding, "These twice a week therapy sessions will be only for about five weeks, I promise, I need to just get everything out on this specific way."

She was thankful for me appreciating her and noticing the time, she took out for me.

There was a time where I would yell at her and take my anger out on her. Nevertheless, she asked me politely to stop months ago, and I did. She did not deserve that, and that rage was not for her. Everything, emotions, and all would turn to deep-seated sorrow, loneliness, and tears beyond streaming tears.

This was a feeling therapy too. The memories had to be separate from the memories. I wanted to hide my emotions in therapy so we would keep going and get the memories out.

Maureen's office was set up perfectly for the work we were doing, she sat across from me and outside the window, and I would stare, and see my spirt animal at the time. The amazing turkey I would exclaim every time I saw one, and Maureen was always happy to see them as well. She used to have a one-eyed small dog that she took out of the pound and would carry it wherever she went.

Maureen was that compassionate.

Her now book became piles of research on my abuse situation. All her print outs sat beside her chair on the floor. She studied, listened, and learned. Above all, she contacted the specialist whenever she needed. By this time, we were moving along and going through each specific issue.

Emotions came out in the office and we had to process because it became too much. I began remembering shameful, unheard of memories that I did not even know were going to come up.

I had my emotional recovery sponsor, Jan. She helped me every day I would call her, cry, sob, sorrow, listen, broken down, and then sheet therapy. Work was not in the picture after I had a nervous breakdown doing retail. I felt like I was going insane until I processed some memories that now were pouring out of me. We all were in a rhythm and ever so slightly if one cord were off or broken, it would bring me to my knees.

In June, it began, Maureen, changed. I saw her disassociating during my session. Staring at the wall, I knew this was not a good sign. We began to argue, because that was my default button.

I already told her and based on last July she knew it was my die month. It was always my worst month, most of the time.

The month of June took a turn I could have never predicted. In the middle of a transition, she made a comment, mean, and I was unable to defend myself because of what I was doing and making changes inside myself and in that moment.

I swung my head back to her, speechless. Maureen looked like a blaze character as well. I do not know what I just did, *what did I just do?* The mark of confusion finally reached her face.

Perplexity reached my facial expression and together it brought the whole session to a halt.

The first thing she said, "Dianne, I am truly sorry, I don't know why I did that to you. That was truly horrible." Then she came clean. "I haven't been feeling right, (meaning with me), and it has been hard to work under this pressure, (meaning with me)."

I could not hold back my disappointment with her and had this incessant need to bring what I have been picking up through her to the forefront, "Maureen, you have been different the last few weeks. I told you July was the worst month for me, so if you think now is bad, July is much worse." I did not nor could not stop, "I can't wait believe what you said to me… I trusted you. But you finally concreted the fact, that all human beings are unreliable."

I froze because I needed her, and knew if I left, it would be the end. I looked at my red memory book; now almost filled to the end from everything we had done in here, from the first memory to the last. She even taught me to have memories and let them go a certain way.

Now she spoke in a less childlike tone, more knowing and assertive but first with, "I am sorry, Dianne, there was no excuse for what I did. I think the changes you see in me is because over the last few weeks, and after we were seeing each other twice a week for a while became really intense, I feel like, dissociated from your abuse—"

Needing to speak, I did, "Maureen this happens to a lot of therapists, it is called something like secondary trauma that the therapist gets. Explaining further, "I had my sponsor I spoke with every day, dying, crying, sobbing, and freaking out every which way. You had nothing, except the specialist."

Maureen still determined, said, "I think I don't know that if that is it. I want you to know that I have and will be talking to the specialist, colleagues, and go online to find support groups for therapists. I just feel that I need to be honest with you too. I feel that how can all this happen. I am not saying I don't believe yo—"

Most definitely it was my turn to speak, "No, that is exactly what you are saying, you're another one that does not believe me, or you cannot take it anymor—"

Now, she was determined, "No that is not what I meant, I do believe you, I hate them, those motherfuckers and what they did to you. Over the last year and a half, I have cried with you, but know I feel differen—"

Now I stopped her before it would be the end I said, "Talk to the specialist, because now, Maureen, YOU need the help, to continue to help me. You are running away in your mind. I am ten steps in front of you, and more of you dissociate. It is normal. Get help or we cannot move forward like this. You call me when you are ready and I will come back, because I do not forget all the kindness, help, and time you gave me. I am loyal, but what you did, damaged me, you need to tell the specialist what you said to me."

By the weekend, Maureen called me.

Hesitantly, I answered, and she began.

"Hello?" was more like a question than anything else was. Feeling unprepared on what I was about to hear.

"Hi Dianne, its Maureen. I wanted to tell you that I spoke with the specialist, my colleagues, join online support groups, and the specialist. She yelled at me for all sorts of things. The support groups were the best; I will tell you more when you come back on Tuesday. There is a lot to tell." Then she asked with trepidation, "Are you coming back Dianne? "

"Yes. I will be there for Tuesday's session." I was honest with her, as I have always been and asked her, "Maureen, how can you be all better in a week and ready to treat me again?"

She said, "Because I get it now, I do believe everything you ever told me, so please don't think it wasn't me not believing you, it was I." She continued, "I joined the support group of therapists and they all said that at one point or another they dissociate too. Now I will be having meetings with them two days a week. It feels so good to have a support group and people who get you." She then said, "Thank You, Dianne."

In disbelief, and wanting to believe she was all better, but not buying it, I replied, "Okay, I am still angry with you so I will be watching you. I do hope you are getting better with this. This is common." I did not want to give her any advice. I knew in my gut, she won this inner conflict, but not truly. It was only a matter of time. I *did* keep this to myself.

"Okay Dianne, I will see you Tuesday, at 10am.

"See you then, Maureen."

I felt differently about her and I needed, we needed to talk more. I just could not end the therapist, client relationship we took a year and a half before building.

Turning this one situation over was more like turning my will and my life over. This point I was on unsteady ground and now I was in uncharted territory. I knew what I felt but I also wanted to believe so badly she would get it back again. Secretly, I thought, I told her too much, now she hates me. As I have hated myself my whole life.

At least there was comfort in knowing I would have my session with her again on Tuesday. Structure was necessary in this recovery. Jan got me through the week. I spoke to my sponsor every day and took her direction. We would argue sometimes, but she always owned it when she was wrong and so would I. I thank her forever, because no matter what I did with Jan, even walk out from her and leave her at a table at the café, screaming at her. She said, "Okay, when you are feeling better, please call me."

With that response to ranting and leaving her there, she took it in, not personal, and kindly asked me to call her. Therefore, I did, time and time again. Glad I did.

Before I knew it, Tuesday had arrived. Jan told me to call her when I was done.

It felt good having her as a backup if there was any fall out form this session.

Maureen came out and got me in the waiting room and she greeted me with happiness. She was almost gleeful. We walked back to her office.

Maureen was shutting the door behind us and said, "Well I feel much better, I am not going to let that happen again." She could not hold it in.

We sat down in our usual chairs.

I peered out the window to my spirit animal out the window. I just sat there waiting for her to start.

She began, and I did not know how much I did not want to be there until she began to speak, "Dianne, the first thing of importance I wanted to say was, I am truly sorry for my actions as a therapist. It was unprofessional to say the least. In addition, I told the specialist exactly what you told me to say to her, I did, and she not only yelled at me for that she yelled at me for other things I said. Dianne, you don't understand, I was on the phone with her for two and a half hours, crying, in disbelief this was happening to me, but I want to tell you the truth,"

Now, I thought, *here it comes.*

Maureen continued, "You said that you were going to kill yourself and I have felt conflicted more and more because you have been saying it more often than usual—"

Now my turn, "I told you July was a horrible month and that I would want to kill myself every day from the pain. You must not have heard me because I am still here and have not killed myself. It helps me just to verbalize it. I don't mean it, or I would have done it years before."

"Well, I do kind of know that, but it is my legal job to report it. So, if it gets much worse, I will have to report it."

She did not need to continue; I knew crap when I saw it.

With sarcasm I said, "Really, this is an excuse. I will not say it again. Now I feel conditioned, but if it makes you feel better, I will not say it again."

Maureen was careful with her words and replied, "Okay, we will not discuss this now, we will see how it goes."

It was weird but I let it slide.

She went back to sounding more upbeat, "The support group I joined as a member will meet twice a week and they all say they have where I have been with the kind of work we have been doing." They gave me tips, some I am not ready to take, but others I am going to try." Reassuring me, "I am still going to go to the support group, and felt good to be understood by women that have been doing this for years and have gone through it, and sometimes it still hits them hard today."

I reassured her, "Maureen, I have told you so much and I know you have had no one to help filter it out so I figured it must have built up." I continued, "The whole time, I have had Jan emotionally available. She has helped me so much. I get it. But you need to stay connect to everyone, because my case is harsh."

She agreed and asked "Dianne, would you like to get started on some therapy right now?"

Swiftly I said, "Yes."

The rest of the session went off without any problems or comments. It felt like we were back to the same duo. Maureen was into it. We accomplished a lot in the time we had left. Ending it on the same way we always do.

"Okay, Dianne. How do you feel?

"Fine"

"Would you like the same time next week?

"Yes. See you next week, Maureen.

We said our good-byes and I left.

Feeling better than when I went into her office, but also feeling, something was not quite right.

A week later, I walked into Maureen's office. Already she had a written up and prepared a monologue for me to say to my doctor. I was not happy; in fact I was downright angry at her.

She took the floor and announced, "Dianne, I have written up a couple paragraphs, (that looked like *War and Peace*). And she continued, It is for you to read this to Timothy."

Automatically, I said, "No."

She tried to convince me because she was worried about me and tried to explain that I said the word, "suicide," one too many times. She began to read it to me. It was bad and I knew I would be sectioned to a mental hospital if I read it to my psychiatrist.

Still, I gave her an unwavering, "No."

I explained to her once again, my side and that I was expressing myself and that the words did not hold any meaning.

Maureen, for some reason, was not having it and said, "We cannot go any further with our work together unless you sign it."

Now, I was in the middle, if I did this, I was going away, and screwed. If I did not do it, I would not trust her again, and felt this was her way of saying that she really was not over what happened to her. I could see it. When all else failed. She pushed me harder.

Which in turn, I rejected.

Therefore, I told her I was not buying what she was selling and that she was not over her trauma. As we did, we got off the topic of calling Timothy.

I asked her, "How is your support doing?"

Answering with her head down, loaded with excuses, saying, well I have the specialist, which is all I needed, I can go back to them when I need them.

Then I flipped the script onto her messed up self and the things she told me in my sessions.

Not mentioning them here will serve her justice because I would be the bigger person.

Eventually, shaken up, Maureen realizes the script is not going to work and had to resort to her written script that I would/or not share with Dr. Holden.

Reiterating back to her what we just did for the whole session, I announced, "So the whole session was wasted, I reminded her. Instead, of working on my issues, which I was coming in with guns blazing and needed to tell you, so many memories. I was deeply saddened by this because I was on the cusp of something insurmountable that I have never reached before and truly a change was severely happening within." Continuing, "I want to thank you for your time on fucking with my head."

I glanced down on the floor where my red book was speaking louder to me. Now I knew, I had to make a decision, in which it would affect me for the rest of my life.

Her eyes widened and she addressed my gestures, "You are not thinking of leaving are you, Dianne?"

Simply, I said, "Yes."

I do not know what ran through her mind, but she was trying so hard to make a deal with me,

"Dianne, why don't you come back on Friday at 11am so we can talk further about this? Maureen asked."

I stated, "I made myself clear are we are going to waste a full session on this? Instead of working on my issues?"

Her eyes rolled up into her forehead, she must have realized how stupid she sounded. She stuck to her stubbornness and said, "Yes, Dianne this is serious. And we have to address it."

In disbelief and at the same time my heart sinking into my stomach. Simultaneously, my heart sank into my stomach and I looked at my red book, one last time.

This time without hesitating, I bent over in my chair, picked it up, and said to Maureen, "Well, I'm done with this stupidity and you not having the guts to end this, I will."

I stood up with all the strength I had left and looked at her.

Now she looking at me in sheer disbelief, her mouth dropped as she said, "You're not leaving are you, Dianne?

As I turned and walked away, I told her, "Yes."

Bolting out the door, hoping she would call me back, she did not. I knew I lost my partner in therapy and help for however long it would take to find another like her, like Patricia. While I walked to my car, I could only ask myself, *"How much time now will it take?" It took me months to find Maureen.*

Now I would have to widen my search, and if needed, I would go to Maine.

Feeling lost and fearing doomed throughout my body. I looked to the sky and asked God for help. I had no more power left in me to search another day, let alone, start this process again with someone I did not know.

My final thought for leaving was, *"Why is this happening to me? Please God, fix this mess."*

12th Therapist
Minnie Mouse

First impressions speak to me the most. Let me write that this woman/girl was barely out of college, which did not serve me well.

Firstly, I had to meet her in the Boston office and she accepted 200.00 as payment. Nevertheless, she did not take any insurances or excuses. Before meeting her in person, we had a zoom meeting on our computers, because it was another two months after Maureen that I had not a drop of therapy and felt like I was going insane with the memories still held deep inside of me. I could not accomplish. It only lasted a week and I made it through my writing, as my red book was finished with, and the new book was not working with me well. I tried with all of my strength, but I needed a professional to take the lead.

I was relying on this therapist/psychologist to help me and I gave her the number of the specialist that worked with Maureen and me.

Minnie Mouse said, "Sure I will call her, but it will only take about fifteen minutes speak with her." With this comment, it meant—troubled waters ahead.

The zoom meeting went well, and she only charged me ninety dollars. *So gracious,* I thought.

But the mouse knew I wanted to work and so she was prepared to do so. I just had to drive through the traffic in Boston during rush hour to see her. I had even asked her, but she was if she could make an exception and schedule a specific time. She said she does it sometimes but just see how it works. I did not like her by the moment.

For the first time I brought Alex. He lived and worked in Boston and knew this part of town. This part of town was weird to begin with, it was the government exit and it just felt wrong. We were early for my appointment, even though we were stuck in traffic for nine hours; we persevered and went for a cup of coffee.

As we were walking around the corner from Minnie Mouse's high-rise office building, I heard a woman, scream from across the street. I turned around behind me and noticed that Alexander was a blob of black, lying face down into the puddle of cement that his face was lost. The woman screaming from across the street came running over and as I was picking him up.

She asked, "Does your friend want to come across the street? I have an office there and plenty of chairs. He is welcome to sit there for as long as he needs."

I looked at him disheveled and immediately we both answered in unison, "No."

Then I said, "Thank you, I am going to grab ice for his head, and he will be okay."

Alex chimed in and backed me up by saying, "Thank you miss, I am okay." Glanced over at me and quickly said, "She will take care of me."

He was scared and I was rather pissed off. Alex always does things like this to mess me up and gain my attention. When I focus on myself.

Alex said, "Dianne, I am sorry, I know how important this meeting is for you and I don't want to mess it up. Maybe I should go to the hospital. I am seeing stars."

As if things could not be any worse.

I looked at his head and sat him down at the end of the fountain.

I said, "I will get you some ice."

He said, "But everything is still closed." Asking, "How will you get a bag of ice?"

Fix-it-up-Dianne responded, "Don't worry. I will be right back with ice for your head."

Jumping into action, I went to a restaurant where everyone was setting up for the lunch shift. My next try was to knock on the door. When I did that. They could not ignore me anymore.

A small woman answered the door and said, "I am sorry miss we do not open until noon."

I replied, "Yes. I know. But my friend, fell and cracked his head open on the concrete right in front of here." Realizing I was shaken up, I continued, "Can I please bother you for a bag of ice? Then I will be out of your hair?"

She glanced over my shoulder at Alex and said, "Absolutely. Come in, I will get you that ice."

Standing in their restaurant with the workers bustling around, I felt bad, embarrassed, now the anger was setting in because Alex does these tricks to have me focus on him and not my health. Secretly, I wanted to kill him, but I was co-dependent with him, I gave up depending on him. Taking Alex anywhere was detrimental to *my* health. I was finally realizing it.

No sooner did I end my conclusion than the worker came out with a huge bag of ice.

She held her hand out and kindly said, "Here, this is for your friend. I hope he feels better."

Taking the bag from her I politely said, "Thank you so much, and this will help him."

She smiled as I walked out the door.

I walked across the street to where the wounded Alexander sat.

He saw me with the bag of ice and exclaimed, "Thank you Dianne, you are amazing!"

Bitterly I replied, "You're welcome."

Even though I was feeling my feelings, I tended to him, and I put the bag on his head and held it there. He was shaking. But he always shook so I was not too worried. Rather, I was worried about getting to my appointment on time.

We had a quick laugh and had to get up, because it was time for my appointment.

He agreed to lean on me as I was hoping I would not run into Minnie in the hallway because she did not know Alexander's attempt to stop this appointment from happening. He was always worried that if I got better, I would leave him. That was not the case. He was my friend. I was loyal to him. The problem was his loyalty came into question the further I went on in recovery. People around me would tell me. Now it was beginning to sink in. Time after time. His attempts to hold me back became obvious.

We made our way to the twentieth floor. It was an over-the-top, modern, glass building. The designers had put frosted glass on them and no sound machines around them. The furniture was cheap and so was this office. To me it was the weirdest office I have been in, as of late.

We waited, hurried up, to wait. It was noon; she was supposed to be here. Unfortunately, she was not. A half an hour passed, Alexander had a dripping bag of water over his head, and my anxiety was through the roof.

Finally, I received a text. It was Minnie Mouse.

The text read, "Hi Dianne, I am stuck at a conference in the government's building, and I am running late. It will be about another half hour before I get there." She knew I drove all the way from Cape Cod just to see her. I was not happy. The traffic only enraged me more but I was so desperate I text her back, "Yes. I will wait."

Her returned text was, "Okay, sit tight, I will be there when I get out. I will run over."

With a simple text, I said, "I will be here. Waiting."

God, this day got worse by the second.

Alexander even grew angry and of course, bad mouthed her. I took the chance to tell him I wanted him dead, everyone, dead. This whole trip was a loss. The sad thing was I believed and had faith that this was my therapist.

Alexander and I did not speak, for what seemed to be an eternity. I kept checking my phone. As Minnie Mouse finally showed up.

She came, one couch as big as a chair, and her chair. In with a cheap necklace, jeans, and a pink sweater. It was all I could do was judge.

Minnie bent down to me as I sat in the one of two chairs and said, "Dianne, I am really sorry."

Then stood up with vigor stating, "I was with the government and I could not leave in the middle of the conference."

From that point on, what I was feeling became a reality, and once I saw that she constantly tried to show me her intelligence—she had none. The Mouse was constantly making up for her insecurity.

We both ran to her cubical and made our way into her claustrophobic room. She told me to sit anywhere. I thought, *really, I had an uninviting couch as small as her chair, where am I going to go?*

Looking to the right of me there was a wall of windows and in front of those windows was the tackiest, long piece of table I had ever seen, gloss and everything.

On top of the table were three modernist open-form sculptures. They were the faces of emotions, like the masks in a play. They were awful. And to top everything off, Minnie's room was painted a turquoise-greenish color, which was my most-hated color.

Then she asked, "So Dianne, what do you think of my office? Do you feel comfortable?"

I figured what was the point of telling her the truth; I already knew I was never going back.

I said, "It is great, I like it."

Sitting so long, I became antsy; I brought my red book in as well as another. To begin working. But she started off with her intelligence, once again.

She said, "I talked to the specialist that worked with you and your last therapist. And I was right; it only took fifteen minutes to know what you guys were doing in therapy."

I did not say one word.

Minnie continued, "The specialist, was good, I have a different way of working—"

I needed to ask, "Have you ever worked with someone with my type of abuse before?"

"I have only once. But I have a lot of experience with other types of abuse."

Telling her, "That is not the same, this is specific."

"Well just try it and the more we get to know each other, the better it will become."

Clearly, I stated, "You said you had an abundance of this kind of experience, but you do not, correct?"

"Well, I have read books that you recommended," she named them.

Again confirming, "They are not the books I recommended."

It became almost an argument and wasting my time was not on my list.

I stopped searching for a therapist because I really thought she could help me. Turns out, I was wrong, and could not understand why my judgment of people has been so off.

Now, I was back to square one.

Looking at the clock, because there was so much rushing, from her.

As she was going with writing, whatever, in her scholarly-of-crap notebook.

She caught me looking at her modernist clock with no numbers and responded, in sarcasm, when she alerted me, "O' do not worry you will get your full time." This did it for me, I knew Minnie, was dumb as dumb could be. The mouse had the appearance of someone that was not nearly strong enough to handle my memories, let alone my emotions.

I could not understand why everyone around me was making light of matters and laughing.

I thought, *wasn't this therapy?*

But I caught on quick, the way people were dressed. It was rich people therapy and they could afford not being truthful, in fact, they probably preferred it that way.

Once I got it, I simply could not sit there one more minute, and said, "Well, I am going to leave now," (more like; make a run for it), this has been a waste of time.

She said, "Well I am sorry this did not work out for you. Sometimes it is just not a good fit for some people."

I knew that was a cut, but I had wasted enough time. It was time to move on fast, do something drastically differently. Nevertheless, the loss of Maureen never left.

Even when Minnie Mouse said, "What your therapist did to you was entirely unprofessional."

Well, what she did was not just bazaar but plain stupidity.

13th Therapist
EMDR to Death

Lisa was not taking any more clients, but she answered my email and agreed to meet with me. We spoke on the phone briefly and she cut her fee in half, still eighty dollars a week, which I knew I could not afford to pay but would figure out some way, because of my desperate need for a therapist, she mentioned all of her EMDR training with a visual machine ready to use with me. Lisa was from the West Coast.

It was one week later, and we agreed to meet. She gave me directions to her house, but I thought as long it was on the Cape it was okay. Traffic alone triggered an emotional reaction. In addition, when I did the EMDR machine with Maureen, it triggered memories.

When I pulled up to Lisa's house. No green in sight. I knocked gently on her door and she had me take my shoes off before entering her house.

We introduced ourselves and had a laugh. She did seem nice enough. However, I could feel her rigidity especially being from the West Coast, she was cold. I did get this feeling that she cared and that is why she took me in as a client. The nervousness about my subject matter seemed to encase us as we walked to her kitchen table where she already had the EMDR machine hooked up.

She explained the machine, as she knew I had experience, it was a brief explanation. Then I gave her my experience with the machine with my former therapist Maureen and that I had read the medical books from Shapiro and other books involving a great many case studies.

Lisa was cool, in terms of she knew I wanted to work. In fact, I was ready for the machine and ready for it to go.

She turned on the EMDR machine, as it looked like Pong, the 1980's video game. This one was visual and within seconds I began my memories on my reel tapes from the computer I built in my mind when I was first sitting up as a baby. In fact, that was the first memory I had. How I built my brain to conquer them and store the tens of thousands of memories. Even as a child, I had the instinct that I would outgrow them. Like everything else, I never knew how anything was going to happen, I just knew, it was going to happen.

With everything stacked against me, and at times even myself, I was able to outsmart the smarties and leave at a young, impressionable age.

After the first vision, or reel, my flashbacks came in incredibly detailed, long slow-moving full memories. Right away, Lisa recorded everything with pencil and paper. It was a lot of information fast. Some parts of the pictures I have had before, now this EMDR machine ran the gamut and people. One of the biggest people in my life back then was my father's brother and my Uncle Louie.

Uncle Louie served on the chief of staff and pioneer at the Children Hospital in Philadelphia, Pennsylvania. Chief of Neuroscience, an inventor, a brilliant man. I began having seizures around six years of age. The family brought me to my uncle's hospital. It was the top children's hospital in the United States. The seizures were grand mal, and I almost died plenty of times. I believe it was from my abuse. The hospital staff took care of the sleep test, all tests, scans, blood work, and everything else. So mechanical. My biological mother acted as if she cared. My father took care of my brother at home. My Uncle Louie came in to check on me from time to time. Sometimes I would stay. While other times I would leave overnight, only to come back again to be poked, prodded, programmed, and the veterans wing of the mental hospital (secretly there) would abuse me. Men with half a brain and face would be on drugs and molest me, or worse. I was powerless. However, they always blamed me. I do not know why but Uncle Louie started to bombard my memories. He taught me a lot about medical science, neuro biology operations, and human behavior. He was a double-sided personality, one split second he would change into his "Evil-Twin." He could change on a dime and only taught me for as long as I was willing. My dad and he had a jealousy. My dad was a hit man, and could sell his way into and out of everything, loudly. Uncle Louie was quieter, smarter in a different way, and wanted my father's kids as his own. He said we were intelligent, not just beautiful.

While his kids had the looks but no brains.

The rivalry between Uncle Louie and my father became more obvious, until the day came when my uncle had a horrible stroke and was only in his mid-forties. It was sad.

Money and power were all that my biological family cared about.

When I would go back, as she did not have this experience, she tried. Lisa read me back my memories from a week ago that triggered me. I never felt like I could be myself around her and I felt judged.

I continued to show up and do the EMDR on a consistent basis. We never processed the memories. I think Lisa was scared to touch them.

As time passed and many memories surfaced, I knew I had to process as I was leaving my emotions by the wayside and myself as well. I was not growing anymore. *Something* had to happen.

Growing angrier at my Lisa, I needed a more emotional connection to process this micro-film of memories.

Once again, I began my long haul of, "Searching for a qualified therapist."

When I told Lisa, I think she was relieved, my intensity of wanting to work seemed overwhelming to her.

We parted on equal terms and no sooner did I reach my car in her driveway than I my phone on the "search therapist" button on my phone.

14th Therapist
The Lazy Girl

Sandy, I thought, could be "The One." Before I went to her office, I spoke on the phone with her and thought *how I could be so lucky, a therapist right around the corner and knowledgeable one too.*

She said, "Dianne, you need to process the memories, as they surface, with emotions and talking about what happened. Not just have them pour out of you and then not process them."

However, the phone call was different from her office. The office seating crowded because she shared the space with twenty other therapists. They had sound machines outside each door, which did not work. With my sensitive hearing, everything amplified into the atmosphere of voices projecting outward. This place was making me even more insane, than before I went there.

When I walked in another therapist gave me a standard form to fill out. Not happy. It was generic again, as an office. Still, I was optimistic as I could be, and was ready to stop searching finding a therapist. Sandy, I thought, was my last hope. But in the back of my mind, I was either going to call Maureen back or go out of state to Maine, because I was hoping to move there anyway.

Sandy's conversation on the telephone with me was enlightening and caring.

She was running late but then she walked through her office door. Sandy was escorting a mentally challenged woman, speaking to her as if she was ten. The Down Syndrome girl was confused, and she had another escort to take her home. I felt bad for her and worse for myself. The good feeling that I had from the phone call grew more silent inside of me. Sandy had a fresh, young, positive outlook on our sessions and that her rent was going to be paid.

Within minutes, the questions she asked stopped with the questions I asked her. Personally, I felt she did not have the experience or determination to see me through a stubbed toenail let alone my issues that were breaking to get out. I mean it felt like they were caged, behind bars and I was circling my prey, desperately trying to work it out. If she did not come up with her lazy girl solution, I was going to come up with something myself because I was so sick of this runaround of crap therapists.

With nowhere else to go, I thought, from our phone call, she gave me a sales call, just to get me on her roster of clients for the weeks ahead.

Asking Sandy, directly, because I got the feeling she was not interested in working, in general.

I asked her, "Sandy, what will you do when I bring up memories?"

Looking perplexed she answered, "I feel in therapy, it is not helpful to bring up your past, your memories."

Now I was perplexed. And thought *what the hell am I here for?*

Then, I threw all my manners out the window, this was in fact survival, and I just existed if I could not purge my memories and get professional guidance.

I reached the end of my rope and said, "Well, Sandy, you cannot be serious. I cannot believe that I wasted my time," I felt the anger rise. Within me and followed my comment with a weird look.

She, like a happy poppy seed, tilted her head and concluded, "Well we believe it is counterproductive and that staying stuck in the past will only cause you more PTSD and you won't work on yourself in the present moment." Sandy then squirmed in her seat, as I looked right through her, I knew she was fully believing her full of shit answers and belief system because as she said, "Well at the university I went to this is the way it is." She was not rude, just idiotic.

About twenty minutes remained on the round, numbered clock between us. The second hand was speaking to me. Saying, *"Get out, Get out." With every second was another Get out."*

Knowing if I waited on more second in that seat, I would lose my life. This was life and death for me and as it turned out it began to be the same outlook for Sandy."

Without another breath of air between us or in the room, I pulled myself out of her pillowed chair and excused myself. Her nervous self ran to her calendar to book me another appointment. Right there and then, as direct as I could have been I said, "No thank you, I have had enough. We believe completely different ways of healing and we are never going to agree."

Before she could plead her case, "But—"

I turned the corner of the office and took off.

Not a minute more.

15th Therapist
The Neuroscientist

Being so down and out, I called Maureen and asked her if she could take me back. Unfortunately, she wanted to take me back and help me again and apologized again but she was leaving Cape Cod to be with her family for good as there was a family emergency. She gave me a referral to a therapist that had helped her for many years. She put in a word for me and told me to call him immediately because he usually does not have any openings.

Doing exactly what she said, no sooner did I leave a message then he called me immediately after. Tom sounded on the phone, knowledgeable, gentle, and kind. We made an appointment in his office over the phone for the following week. It made me feel safe knowing I was in a real professional's hands. Maureen, again was by the wayside.

Next week came and our appointment had arrived. I was early with anticipation. He and his client came out of his session and he kindly told me to hold on for one minute. The client said goodbye to him, and he went into a back office. My guess to exhale and gain perspective for me, his new client.

In the waiting room, which was beautiful, costly, and tasteful. Now this waiting room was friendly and had updated magazines such as: *Time* Magazine, *New York Times Book Review*, *National Geographic*, and many others. The furniture itself was antique with a modern element of style.

Then Tom came out of his back office in a cashmere baby blue sweater with a soft patterned dress shirt underneath. He was a fine dresser in his unassuming ways.

He could see I was nervous, stood far back from me as he spoke softly to me, guided me with his hand as he welcomed me, and pointed to his therapy office.

I took his cue and swiftly moved into the room as I took the furthest seat from him on the couch across from him. Automatically, I was four again looking for answers to the happenings that caused me pain. He did slow me down as I wanted and needed to work everything out that minute. The moment he slowed me down I was able to gather myself and saw his discomfort. His actions to me were one of a weak person. He clammed up and crossed his legs and his arms, simultaneously. I let that go for now but not without asking a question.

I asked, "So, please explain to me how this will work for you and me. I do not want to spend time not working. Maureen said you taught her, you obviously have a lot of experience and degrees but deep down, what is your therapeutic process?" Adding, "Do you believe that I should have memories from the past or just forget the past and move on?" Continuing, "I think I need to get to the bottom of everything, learn, and grow from it."

He responded first with his body language; by crossing his legs the other way and refolding his hands tenser as his face became more flushed.

His answer, "Firstly, I think we should get to know you, and then if anything comes out, we will process it as it goes."

That was the final nail. The big IF again. Now it meant to me as a warning sign, almost not to have my memories.

In his quiet demeanor, he demanded an agreement. I complied with a simple and stunned, "Yes."

My first thought was, *well maybe he was right. I mean he helped Maureen.*

My second though was, *start looking for a place and therapist in Maine.*

I felt it in my heart and throughout my gut. This was not going to work in the end but he would work for a couple of months so I could look and find a real therapist.

As he talked about his process of going from Yale to Hale, my eyes and mind drifted of out his window and laid their sight upon the trees and all nature outside. Wishing someday, I could be as free as they could. It has been a long haul, but I was not giving up the fight. I would do the work, the next right thing, and let my Higher Power lead me. Then I focused my attention back into the room as he said, "How does that sound to you, Dianne."

I felt like telling him the truth but instead, I parroted back to him, "Okay, Sounds good."

He was male and weird. Tom reminded me of a voyager with his patients. He WAS the white Milton.

I found the commonality of neuroscience and neuropsychology as my artwork and essays were evolving into that subject matter. He was excited that I was interested in this and we mostly talked about these topics in the months that he was my therapist.

At least I found an intelligent person to banter back and forth about the brain, books, and other subjects that interest me.

My seat would get closer to him on the couch. As I felt more comfortable in his strangeness. I had my own weirdness to contend with, so I stopped, for the most part, judging him.

He kept exclaiming the phrases, "Dianne, you know more neuroanatomy than me, and more neuroscience as well, it is wonderful to speak with you about interesting things!"

Then he would say, "I think you're a genius. You have so much intelligence and you are so knowledgeable, yet curious all the while."

The sessions were just to talk shop now.

Occasionally, I gave him a memory and feelings, tears, sorrow, and the bewilderment of betrayal. He would cry with me. Then explained that his tears were purely out of empathy. Tom a look of shock on his face too.

Nevertheless, I then would switch back to the subject matter that he could endure. I figured; I have endured this pain for so long that I can handle it. That is when I actively took the steps on the website to look for a Maine therapist. None took insurance, their sliding scale was more like a slippery slope into debt BUT they did have some good therapists. This meant... I would be moving there.

This is when I broke the news to Tom, about moving to Maine for a quieter life and finding another therapist up there. I told him I did not know how long it would take but I would keep my sessions with him but since my lease was running out, I needed to move fast and find someone up there.

Besides, Tom had a hearing aid and every time I would stop talking and asked him a question, he was completely lost, even though he was nodding his head.

The whole three months I have been talking to a deaf therapist.

Then Covid-19 hit, everyone flew into fear, which was understandable, at the time. Tensions arose and now doctors including Thomas worked at home on a video chat. There were delays and it was even harder for him to hear me. Half the session I had to repeat my words to him because he could not read my lips.

I knew it was time to cut the cord. First I went to a therapist in Maine, before Covid-19 hit as bad as it would. She is not even worth giving a few sentences worth. She was out for the money and I drove up in an ice storm for a twelve-hour drive, which would usually take two hours. That was that.

Back to Thomas, I told him my experience and told him I needed to fast-forward my life into action and change this story. It was time for me to move on. I felt it.

In the end, he was disappointed but kind and generous by saying, "Dianne, if you ever want to come back here for therapy, please call me."

Thomas was a good person. Those are hard to find. I did wind up cherishing what we had.

16th Therapist
The Maine Therapist

This one could be the one. As Covid-19 grew worse in the entire world. Alaina and I managed to schedule regular therapy through internet sessions and from day one, while I was still living on the Cape, she got me. We were working from my cottage on Cape Cod to her house in Maine. She totally cut the cost of her sessions because she was a true humanitarian who cared about her clients and people in general.

Alaina was strong and steady. She had boundaries and always explained the reason why she did not want me or anyone for that matter to get therapist dependent. She had over thirty-five-years' experience.

Naturally, I had to ask, "Does that mean you are going to retire? I finally get a good therapist who knows how to work with me and read me. Then you are going to drop me?"

She intervened, "I am going to be around for you for a few years. Dianne, I thought long and hard about the work we would have to do to get you into a good place. I decided to work with you because you have done a lot of the work and you are fearless when it comes to meeting, your issues, then, when you are settled, I would get you the right therapist I know and will guide you from there."

Our first meeting she nailed down the toughest part of my childhood self and she got it. It was as if I surrendered and could not fight anymore. I began to let go of the guilt, even though she told me it was not my fault, I believed, everything was my fault. It was as a hundred-pound bag of rocks flung over my shoulders that I needed to put down, finally rest and sit by the side of the road and, for once, view my life. Reality. It was sad; she hit the true sorrow Maureen left off. It all came flooding back.

Once a week we met like clockwork. Always online, as the pandemic grew to an impossible level.

I knew she was good before we even properly met. Alaina wanted to talk to Maureen, the last real person I did this heavy-duty work with and take it from there. Maureen, of course, agreed.

After Alaina spoke with her little details of their conversations would come out and the biggest thing was that she understood it but also wanted me to trust her because she had her own way of working with me. She was another well-educated therapist that had a PhD at an Ivy League school.

I asked her, "Alaina how you pick up on things and the toughest issues came up first and you are great at picking up on my subtleties?"

She answered, "Well, Dianne, I usually listen to what is happening with you that week, at first. Then I pick up a thread throughout what you are telling me and follow you in the tread and treat you accordingly." She added, "But you are not easy to follow, you do go all over the place, because your mind is working in overdrive, I slow you down, then I lead you or you lead me to what is really happening in your core self."

Stunned, my reply to her was, "That is some way to put it. It is both logical and rational." I continued, "You are definitely one of the best if not the best therapist I've had."

Alaina took the compliment well. She put her hand over her chest, took a deep breath, and gasp, then said, "Well you are a good client and willing to work on yourself no matter how bad the pain gets. That is why I am willing to help you. Maureen said a lot of great things about you and your character and only wanted the best for you."

Our conversation flowed to the end of the session.

As Covid-19 began to exacerbate, Alaina and I were continuingly meeting once a week, having memories, the deepest, and processing to the degree I never have before. Now realizing the work I did with Patricia and Maureen, opened me up to this type of depth on working on myself. As I became more centered, I continued, with Alaina, as I felt she had the right answers and really did allow me to pay on a sliding scale. She cared and believed me, which was the most important thing of all.

She was honest and had no hidden agenda. She was an old-fashioned therapist with a PhD. I trusted her, she would make sure I knew that she would hear me and work for me to get me better and grow, out of therapy and into life.

Which is what I always wanted. I have always been misunderstood, eccentric, and crazy at times. At my best, nothing can touch me. I knew Alaina could bring me there if given the chance. She really was my last hope.

The problem was to be open, honest, and not a pain. I never felt the urge to be mean to her or abusive. She took my case with a lot of thought, care, and experience. Maureen continued her education and remained curious throughout our sessions.

The gratitude I feel for her helping me is beyond immense.

I still keep her words of wisdom, along with Patricia's, in my mind.

Learning to be silent, not reacting, and continuing to grow is my straightforward path.

No matter what, if I survived my childhood the first time around as well as living on the streets by the age of eight. Asking God for help, doing the next right thing, staying present were and still are the lessons I have learned from my teachers. If the same "problem" or scenario occurs, it is up to me to continue to live, not worry about what anyone else thinks, even their lies, ridicule, and shame. I am all the better for it.

Because it has nothing to do with me. I am not running anymore. Or having expectations. I have learned human beings are fallible and flawed as well.

Harboring any type of resentment, bitterness, or ill will is not welcome anymore. Only peace, helping others, and not losing light on myself, mentally, emotionally, physically, and spiritually.

I welcome the future and say goodbye to the past.